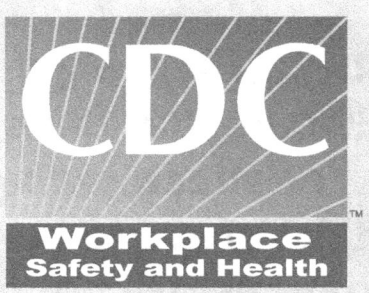

I0426400

Evaluation of Exposures to Pesticides and Parasitic Vectors During Inspection of Imported Aquatic Plants

Srinivas Durgam, MSPH, MSChE, CIH
Carlos Aristeguieta, MD, MPH

Health Hazard Evaluation Report
HETA 2008-0070-3112
U.S. Department of Agriculture
Animal and Plant Health Inspection Service
Los Angeles, California
July 2010

Department of Health and Human Services
Centers for Disease Control and Prevention

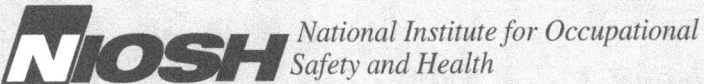

National Institute for Occupational Safety and Health

CONTENTS

ABBREVIATIONS

μg	Microgram
μg/m³	Micrograms per cubic meter of air
ACGIH®	American Conference of Governmental Industrial Hygienists
APHIS	Animal and Plant Health Inspection Service
BHC	Benzene hexachloride
CDC	Centers for Disease Control and Prevention
CFR	Code of Federal Regulations
DDD	Dichlordiphenyldichloroethane
DDE	Dichlorodiphnyldichloroethylene
DDT	Dicholordiphenyltrichloroethane
EPA	Environmental Protection Agency
FOH	Federal Occupational Health
GA	General area
HHE	Health hazard evaluation
LOD	Limit of detection
MDC	Minimum detectable concentration
NAICS	North American Industry Classification System
NIOSH	National Institute for Occupational Safety and Health
OEL	Occupational exposure limit
OSHA	Occupational Safety and Health Administration
PBZ	Personal breathing zone
PEL	Permissible exposure limit
PPE	Personal protective equipment
PPQ	Plant Protection and Quarantine
REL	Recommended exposure limit
SOP	Standard operating procedure
STEL	Short term exposure limit
TLV®	Threshold limit value
TWA	Time-weighted average
USDA	U.S. Department of Agriculture
WEEL	Workplace environmental exposure level

Highlights of the NIOSH Health Hazard Evaluation

The National Institute for Occupational Safety and Health (NIOSH) received a health hazard evaluation request from a management representative of the U.S. Department of Agriculture, Animal and Plant Health Inspection Service (APHIS) in Riverdale, Maryland. The requestor was concerned about potential hazards from inspecting imported aquatic plants at Plant Protection and Quarantine stations throughout the United States. No health effects among APHIS employees were listed in the request.

What NIOSH Did

- We evaluated the Los Angeles Plant Protection and Quarantine station in September–October 2008.

- We observed the plant inspection process, employee work practices, and personal protective equipment use.

- We tested the air and work surfaces for pesticides.

- We talked to employees about their work and health.

- We reviewed a previous surface wipe sampling report, injury and illness records, and standard operating procedures.

What NIOSH Found

- We did not detect pesticides in the air or on surfaces. Because of these findings, we did not identify a need for respiratory protection during routine plant inspections.

- Some employees tried to detect pesticides on the plants by smelling them.

- The written respiratory protection program required the use of respirators for specific tasks such as welding and fumigation. However, the program did not provide guidance for worksite-specific procedures such as the chemical dip process.

- Employees regularly wore disposable gloves when inspecting imported plants.

- Employees did not report work-related symptoms. They were aware of the potential hazards from disease-carrying insects and snails found in aquatic plant shipments.

- We found no recorded injuries or illnesses.

- Inspecting imported aquatic plants poses a potential risk of parasitic and bacterial infection.

What Managers Can Do

- Revise the written respiratory protection program to provide worksite-specific guidance. The written program should identify job tasks and job locations that require respiratory protection and note the level of protection.

- Include the list of disease-carrying snails in the APHIS Safety and Health Manual. This list should be updated periodically.

- Communicate any changes that are made to standard operating procedures and other written materials that guide employees in their daily job duties. These changes should be shared with employees through written and oral communication.

What Employees Can Do

- Continue to wear disposable gloves and use absorbent pads such as newspapers when inspecting imported plants.

- Do not smell the plants for pesticides during inspection.

- Wash hands thoroughly prior to eating, drinking, smoking, and after removing gloves.

- Wear a face shield along with safety glasses and long sleeve lab coats if work activities pose a splash hazard.

NIOSH received a management request to evaluate employee exposures during inspection of imported aquatic plants. None of the 20 pesticides that were analyzed for were detected in air or on surfaces. Employees did not report work-related health symptoms. We recommend that employees continue to use PPE such as disposable gloves and long sleeve lab coats when inspecting imported plants.

In January 2008, NIOSH received an HHE request from a management representative of the USDA APHIS in Riverdale, Maryland. The requestor was concerned about potential hazards from aquatic plant inspections conducted at PPQ stations throughout the United States. No health effects among APHIS employees were listed in the request. The APHIS PPQ station in Los Angeles, California, was chosen for evaluating exposure risks resulting from disease-carrying insects and pesticides because it has a high volume and frequency of imported aquatic plant shipments.

On September 29–October 3, 2008, we made a site visit to the APHIS PPQ station in Los Angeles, California. We met with management and employee representatives and observed work processes, practices, and workplace conditions. We collected PBZ air samples and surface wipe samples to evaluate pesticide exposures. We talked to employees about their work and related symptoms. We reviewed APHIS wipe sampling records, the OSHA Form 300 Log of Work-Related Injuries and Illnesses for 2005–2008, and other pertinent records.

We did not detect the 20 pesticides we analyzed for in the air or on surface wipe samples. No work-related symptoms among APHIS PPQ inspectors were reported. Our findings indicated that respiratory protection is not needed during routine inspection of imported plants. The written respiratory protection program required respirators for specific tasks such as welding and fumigation. However, the program lacked guidance for worksite-specific procedures such as the chemical dip process, and employees were uncertain about when respirators were needed. Employees used disposable gloves when conducting plant inspections and knew the potential hazards from disease-carrying insects found in aquatic plant shipments. We found a potential risk of contracting a parasitic or bacterial infection from splashes with contaminated water when inspecting aquatic plants.

We recommend revising the written respiratory protection program to provide worksite-specific guidance including the type of respirator needed and job tasks that require respirator use. Employees should continue to wear disposable gloves, clear face shields along with safety glasses, and long sleeve garments such as lab coats to further minimize the potential for inadvertent exposure to pesticides and disease-carrying insects. Employees should also continue to use newspapers or other absorbent pads to absorb residual contaminated water when inspecting imported aquatic plants.

Keywords: NAICS 926140 (Regulation of Agricultural Marketing and Commodities), plant inspection, aquatic plants, snails, pesticides, PPE

INTRODUCTION

In January 2008, NIOSH received an HHE request from a management representative of the USDA APHIS in Riverdale, Maryland. The requestor was concerned about potential hazards from aquatic plant inspections conducted at PPQ stations throughout the United States, specifically contact with pesticides and disease-carrying snails and insects. No health effects among APHIS employees were listed in the request. Plant inspections are conducted at APHIS PPQ stations throughout the United States. The APHIS PPQ station in Los Angeles, California, was chosen as a suitable site for evaluating exposure risks resulting from disease-carrying insects and pesticides because it has a high volume and frequency of imported aquatic plant shipments.

On September 29–October 3, 2008, we made a site visit to the APHIS PPQ station in Los Angeles, California. We met with management and employee representatives and observed work processes, practices, and workplace conditions. We also spoke with employees about their work and whether they experienced symptoms they related to workplace exposures. We collected PBZ air samples and surface wipe samples to evaluate pesticide exposures. We held a closing conference with management and employee representatives on October 3, 2008, to summarize site visit activities and provide preliminary recommendations.

Background

USDA APHIS is responsible for protecting U.S. agriculture from foreign pests and diseases. APHIS PPQ employees inspect imported cut flowers (roses, chrysanthemums, carnations, etc.), produce (fruit and vegetables), and live plants (dry land and aquatic). The objectives of the imported commodity inspections are to ensure that plants and produce are free of disease and infestation (snails, insects, and noxious weeds) and are not an endangered or threatened species. This inspection is required prior to releasing the products into U.S. trade markets. APHIS PPQ inspectors not only look for plant diseases, but also for vectors of human diseases, and can serve as quarantine personnel. Aquatic plants arrive in the United States through five main port cities, with the largest quantity of aquatic plant shipments arriving through Los Angeles, Seattle, and Miami. The APHIS PPQ facilities in these cities reportedly ranged from antiquated to state-of-the-art, although plans are in place to build new facilities to replace old ones, including the Los Angeles facility.

Aquatic plants are imported from nurseries all over the world. Plants can come from state-of-the-art USDA-certified facilities or from brackish backyard ponds. Review of aquatic plant shipment inspection records from January 1–December 31, 2007, indicated that shipments arrived from Southeast Asian countries such as Singapore, Thailand, and Indonesia, as well as Costa Rica, the Netherlands, and Guatemala. Exporters are not required to label or provide information about whether a plant shipment has been treated with a pesticide.

Seven inspectors (four full-time and three part-time) worked at the PPQ station in Los Angeles during our evaluation. The standard inspection service is from 8:00 a.m. to 4:30 p.m., Monday through Friday. Because of the perishable nature of the imported material, on-call service is available 24 hours a day, including weekends. PPQ inspectors and management representatives constitute a five-person health and safety committee.

Plant Protection and Quarantine Inspection Process

Import brokers bring the plants to the PPQ facility for inspection. When an imported plant shipment arrives, U.S. Customs and Border Protection personnel issue a provisional release to the importers on the condition that the plants are approved by the PPQ inspectors. The import broker or freight forwarder then initiates the request for an inspection. Inspection time per shipment ranges from 30 minutes to 1 hour depending on the size of the shipment and experience with the particular commodity (a representative sample of the shipment is inspected). Daily logs note the size of the shipment, plant type, country of origin, and the name of the exporter. During inspections, there is considerable handling of the plants, including vigorous shaking of the plants over an examination table to dislodge insects and snails onto the examination table. Aquatic plants are mostly individually packaged and are kept moist to prevent plants from perishing during transit. Plants suspected of disease upon initial visual examination are closely examined using a magnifying glass; samples are collected and examined further under a stereo microscope by the PPQ inspector, who may take the sample to a biologist for confirmation. After passing inspection, the plants are released to the importer. If a shipment does not pass inspection (insect infestation or plant disease is detected), the broker has the option of returning the

INTRODUCTION
(CONTINUED)

entire shipment to the country of origin, destroying the plants in a gas-fired incinerator, treating the plants offsite at a methyl bromide fumigation station, or treating the infestation at the PPQ station using appropriate chemicals. The on-site treatment of plants is referred to as a "chemical dip" process.

At the Los Angeles PPQ station, PPQ inspectors oversee contractors responsible for cargo fumigation as well as brokers conducting on-site treatment using the chemical dip process.

Previous NIOSH HHEs

In 1995–1996, NIOSH investigators conducted two evaluations at the APHIS PPQ station in Miami, Florida, to evaluate the potential for employee exposure to pesticides during inspection of imported plants. Both evaluations found pesticide residue on foliage and determined that PPQ inspectors were at risk for skin exposure to pesticides. Pesticides were not detected in air samples collected during either evaluation; therefore, respiratory protection was not recommended. Disposable glove use was recommended at all times during inspection. The investigators concluded that human senses such as smell and presence of visible residue should not be used to determine whether PPE should be worn [NIOSH 1997a, 1997b].

ASSESSMENT

We observed the inspection process for imported plants, noted PPE availability and use, and observed housekeeping practices. PPQ inspectors inspected aquatic plants on October 2 and 3, 2008. Imported plants can contain a variety of residual pesticides, the specifics of which are not known to PPQ inspectors [NIOSH 1997a, 1997b]. Therefore, our air and surface wipe samples were analyzed for 20 common pesticides, including isomers of these compounds, using a gas chromatograph with a mass spectrometer detector according to EPA Method TO-10A. Chromatogram peaks for all the eluted chemicals were also identified and their identities confirmed from the spectral library. We collected seven PBZ and five GA full-shift air samples to assess pesticide exposure during the plant inspection process. We also collected 15 surface wipe samples for pesticides, including 13 from three work tables and two from high contact surfaces (the viewfinder and focusing knobs of two different microscopes). Details on the air and surface

ASSESSMENT
(CONTINUED)

wipe sampling methods used in this evaluation are described in Appendix A; a discussion of occupational exposure limits and health effects for pesticides is in Appendix B.

We interviewed employees informally about symptoms that may have been related to their workplace exposure and any concerns about workplace exposures. We also reviewed the following documents:

- Industrial hygiene report assessing the presence of pesticides in plant shipments at the San Juan airport conducted by FOH, dated May 14, 2008

- OSHA Form 300 Log of Work-related Injuries and Illnesses from 2005–2008 for the Los Angeles facility

- SOP for the chemical dip process

- APHIS Safety and Health Manual, current version dated 2004

- Circular and memorandum from CDC to USDA listing snails of medical importance [Ciordano 1972; Sullivan 1990].

We consulted with a parasitologist from the CDC National Center for Zoonotic, Vector-Borne, and Enteric Diseases, who also serves as a subject matter expert for APHIS. He confirmed that he was not aware of any reports of adverse health effects among APHIS PPQ inspectors and that he has had previous discussions with APHIS personnel about aquatic snails found in shipments from Southeast Asia and Peru [Sullivan 2008]. He created a list of aquatic snails with potential for transmitting parasitic diseases that was shared with APHIS in May 1998. This list has not been updated since 1998.

RESULTS

None of the 20 pesticides we analyzed for were detected in PBZ and GA air samples or in surface wipe samples. The MDC for the 20 pesticides whose concentrations were quantitatively determined in the air samples are presented in Appendix A. The analytical LODs for pesticides analyzed in the surface wipe samples are also listed in Appendix A. Captan 50 W, a fungicide, was qualitatively identified in one of the air samples at an estimated concentration of 1.5 µg/m³.

Although APHIS PPQ inspectors have reported no work-related illnesses (specifically no parasitic disease, insect bites, or pesticide intoxication), they have observed snails, insects, and visible residue on some plant shipments and were concerned about contaminated residual water arriving with aquatic plant shipments. No aquatic snails were found on aquatic plants during our evaluation. The OSHA Logs also listed no injuries or illnesses.

Document Review

The FOH report from the San Juan PPQ station included three wipe samples, two from orchid leaves and one from the inside of a cardboard box. The samples were analyzed for organophosphorous pesticides and for Captan. Captan, a fungicide, ranged from 10–170 µg/sample and chlorpyrifos, an organophosphorus insecticide, ranged from not detected to 0.11 µg/sample. No other organophosphorous pesticides were detected. FOH recommended conducting personal air sampling for pesticides identified in its evaluation.

The written SOP for the chemical dip process required the brokers to use safety goggles, nitrile gloves, protective long sleeve clothing, and respirators when using specific pesticides. A "NIOSH-approved cartridge respirator" was to be used when using Sevin® or malathion, and a "respirator mask" was required when using "Bordeaux" fungicide. No additional details on the specific type of respirator or respirator cartridges were provided.

The APHIS Safety and Health Manual described testing programs for pesticides and communicable diseases of public health concern. The PPE section described jobs "typically requiring respiratory protection include laboratory work, welding, cutting or brazing, handling hazardous chemicals or substances, and during pesticide application or fumigation" [Petch 2008]. The written respiratory protection program section governs all APHIS facilities in the United States and discusses evaluating operations to determine the nature of the hazard and level of respiratory protection needed, selection of respirators, employee training, medical requirements, fit testing, and maintenance of respirators.

The two CDC documents together list approximately 100 aquatic snails that can act as hosts for a dozen parasites of public health importance. The documents state that aquatic plant shipments contaminated with snails of public health importance should be treated with a molluscicide, incinerated, or returned to the broker.

Other Observations and Findings

The Los Angeles APHIS management informed us that PPQ inspectors were provided with lab coats to prevent transfer of contamination from agricultural products to their uniforms. However, we found no lab coats in the inspection area, and PPQ inspectors were not aware of their availability.

PPQ inspectors wore disposable latex or nitrile gloves that were typically discarded after each inspection. Dry products were laid on the inspection benches for examination; however, when inspecting aquatic plants, the inspectors covered benches with newspaper to absorb any condensate present in the shipment. These newspapers were disposed of after each inspection. PPQ inspectors informed us that they used bleach on alternate days to clean work surfaces before starting their work shift. PPQ inspectors used a long brush and a dust pan to clean surfaces between shipment inspections. We observed some PPQ inspectors checking for pesticides on the plants by smelling them.

Although we did not observe the chemical dip process during our site visit, PPQ inspectors explained the process to us. At the Los Angeles PPQ station, the process is conducted by the broker after normal business hours in a separate room fitted with a wall mounted exhaust fan. The pesticide is diluted to the required concentration in large wide-mouth tubs. Infected plant material is dipped completely in the solution and then air dried on shelves in the room. The broker is responsible for obtaining all the required PPE per the APHIS written SOP for this process. PPQ inspectors in the area during this process have the potential of being exposed to pesticides used for treating plant shipments.

Neither respiratory protection nor special clothing are required during routine plant inspections. However, activities such as shaking wet plants can pose a splash hazard against which employees need to be adequately protected. We noted that PPQ inspectors were provided one air-purifying elastomeric half-mask respirator equipped with a combination organic vapor and P100 particulate filter (North by Honeywell, Cranston, Rhode Island)

RESULTS

for common use. PPQ inspectors mentioned that they were fit tested for this respirator but were unclear about its intended use. In addition, APHIS provided no air monitoring results that would support the need for respiratory protection. PPQ inspectors used the respirator voluntarily; its use was rare because the broker, with guidance from PPQ inspectors, conducted the chemical dip process. In addition, PPQ inspectors had not received a copy of Appendix D of the OSHA respiratory protection standard (29 CFR 1910.134), which is required when employees voluntarily use respirators.

DISCUSSION

Pesticides typically have a high molecular weight and are nonvolatile compounds. The highest exposures to pesticides have been reported in workers handling and/or applying pesticides during farming activities [Curwin et al. 2005]. Pesticide exposures can occur through ingestion, skin contact, and inhalation. However, in occupational settings, worker exposure occurs primarily through skin contact and to a lesser extent by inhalation [Geno et al. 1996; Franklin and Worgan 2005]. The aquatic plant shipments we observed contained plants individually wrapped in plastic with some residual moisture usually present.

According to EPA, more than 1055 active ingredients are registered as pesticides, which are formulated into thousands of pesticide products [EPA 2007]. All these compounds cannot be sampled and analyzed using a single analytical method. We used EPA Method TO-10A with gas chromatography-mass spectroscopy analysis to confirm the identity of chemical compounds in the air and in surface wipe samples. We detected none of the 20 pesticides we specifically analyzed for in our air samples. However, using mass spectroscopy we identified the presence of Captan 50 W, a fungicide, in one air sample. The chemical dip process was not conducted during the time of our evaluation; therefore, we could not evaluate PPQ inspectors' exposures during this task.

We found none of the 20 pesticides we analyzed for in the 18 surface wipe samples. However, PPQ inspectors may be splashed with the residual water in aquatic plant shipments when they vigorously shake the plants. No pesticide surface contamination standards exist, but the presence of surface contamination can indicate the need for improved housekeeping and the potential for dermal exposure or ingestion from contaminated hands, clothing, or work surfaces.

In their natural habitat, aquatic plants can harbor insects and snails that serve as vectors for parasitic diseases. For example, eosinophilic meningitis, a presentation of infection with the parasite *Angiostrongylus cantonensis*, can be contracted by skin contact with or ingestion of infected aquatic snails of the genus *Pila* sp. Although the risk of infection is greatest for people living and working in areas where these plants are grown, APHIS inspectors are at risk of accidental contact with these insects and snails. In addition, aquatic plants may be grown in water contaminated with human or animal feces, which may carry disease-causing bacteria. When inspecting shipments of aquatic plants, APHIS inspector's skin and mucosa could be exposed to potentially contaminated water [Rosen 1998]. APHIS inspectors were aware of the hazards associated with exposure to snails and contaminated water in aquatic plant shipments. To reduce this possibility of exposure, they regularly wear disposable gloves. Although this exposure awareness exists, the inspectors do not use lab coats or eye or face protection when inspecting aquatic plants.

Although the APHIS written respiratory protection program has most elements of a comprehensive respiratory protection program, it lacks guidance for worksite-specific procedures. For example, it does not provide specific guidance on the type of respirator the broker should use during the chemical dip process. PPQ inspectors had access to one respirator and indicated that it was available for common use if needed, but did not know the intended use (i.e., under what conditions). This suggests a gap in employee training and a lack of site-specific implementation of the respiratory protection program.

The written SOP for the chemical dip process did not provide specific PPE guidance. Nitrile gloves are appropriate when using carbaryl (brand name Sevin®) but are not appropriate for use with malathion. Silver Shield® gloves are recommended when using malathion [Forsberg and Mansdorf 2007]. Tighter fitting gloves such as disposable nitrile gloves should be worn over the Silver Shield gloves to increase dexterity.

CONCLUSIONS

We conclude that no health hazard to pesticides existed for APHIS personnel conducting plant inspections. Our findings indicate that no respiratory protection is needed during routine inspection of imported plants. Contracting a parasitic or bacterial infection from inspecting imported aquatic plants is a potential risk. However, a clean work environment, regular PPE use, and low frequency of aquatic plant shipments make this an unlikely event. Disposable gloves, long sleeve garments such as lab coats, and face shields along with safety glasses will help prevent employee exposure to pesticides, parasites, bacteria, and disease-carrying insects that may be present in imported plant shipments.

RECOMMENDATIONS

Based on our findings, we recommend the actions listed below to create a more healthful workplace. We encourage APHIS to use the existing labor-management health and safety committee to discuss the recommendations in this report and develop an action plan. Those involved in the work can best set priorities and assess the feasibility of our recommendations for the specific situation at APHIS PPQ station in Los Angeles, California. Our recommendations are based on the hierarchy of controls approach (Appendix B: Occupational Exposure Limits and Health Effects). This approach groups actions by their likely effectiveness in reducing or removing hazards. In most cases, the preferred approach is to eliminate hazardous materials or processes and install engineering controls to reduce exposure or shield employees. Until such controls are in place, or if they are not effective or feasible, administrative measures and/or personal protective equipment may be needed.

Administrative Controls

Administrative controls are management-dictated work practices and policies to reduce or prevent exposures to workplace hazards. The effectiveness of administrative changes in work practices for controlling workplace hazards is dependent on management commitment and employee acceptance. Regular monitoring and reinforcement are necessary to ensure that control policies and procedures are not circumvented in the name of convenience or production.

1. Revise the written respiratory protection program to identify the job tasks, type of respirator, and work locations where

respirator use is required. Respiratory hazards should be evaluated for job tasks where respiratory protection is currently required to ensure that the respirators worn are necessary and appropriate. If respirators are deemed necessary, the respirator program must identify the type of respirator required for those tasks (e.g., chemical dip process). Job tasks where employees may voluntarily wear respirators should also be noted in the written program. Ensure that the requirements listed in the OSHA Respiratory Protection Standard (29 CFR 1910.134) are followed. The OSHA *Small Entity Compliance Guide* provides guidance for respiratory protection programs and is available at http://www.osha.gov/Publications/SECG_RPS/secg_rps.html.

2. Revise the SOP for the chemical dip process to specify the user and the type of respirator to be worn, if needed.

3. Instruct employees not to smell the plants in an attempt to detect the presence of pesticides during inspection.

4. Encourage employees to wash hands with soap and water before eating, drinking, smoking, and after removing gloves.

5. Communicate to employees in writing any changes that are made to SOPs and other written materials that guide them in their daily job duties.

6. Integrate the list of disease-carrying snails into the APHIS Safety and Health Manual. The list should be periodically reviewed and updated by CDC's medical parasitologist.

Personal Protective Equipment

PPE is the least effective means for controlling employee exposures. Proper use of PPE requires a comprehensive program, and calls for a high level of employee involvement and commitment to be effective. The use of PPE requires the choice of the appropriate equipment to reduce the hazard and the development of supporting programs such as training, change-out schedules, and medical assessment if needed. PPE should not be relied upon as the sole method for limiting employee exposures. Rather, PPE should be used until engineering and administrative controls can be demonstrated to be effective in limiting exposures to acceptable levels.

RECOMMENDATIONS
(CONTINUED)

1. Continue to wear appropriate disposable gloves, preferably nonlatex, when routinely inspecting imported plant shipments. Some employees exposed to latex products such as latex gloves can develop latex allergy. Additional information on latex allergy and related hazards is available at http://www.cdc.gov/niosh/topics/latex/.

2. If inspecting aquatic plants poses a potential splash hazard, wear clear face shields along with safety glasses and long sleeve garments such as lab coats.

3. Continue to use newspapers as absorbent pads or procure disposable absorbent pads for use when inspecting imported aquatic plants.

4. Wear tighter fitting disposable nitrile gloves over the Silver Shield gloves when using a mixture of sevin and malathion insecticides in the chemical dip process.

REFERENCES

Ciordano JF [1972]. Circular No. 132 (Revised) Supplement 2 of December 11, 1972, from J.F. Giordano, Quarantine Program, Epidemiology Program, to Officers in Charge, Type I and II Quarantine Stations, Centers for Disease Control, U.S. Department of Health, Education and Welfare.

Curwin BD, Hein MJ, Sanderson WT, Barr DB, Heederik D, Reynolds SJ, Ward EM, Alavanaja MC [2005]. Urinary and hand wipe pesticide levels among farmers and nonfarmers in Iowa. J Expo Anal Environ Epidemiol 15(6):500–508.

EPA [2007]. Assessing health risks from pesticides. [http://www.epa.gov/pesticides/factsheets/ riskassess.htm]. Date accessed: April 2010.

Forsberg K, Mansdorf SZ [2007]. Quick selection guide to protective clothing. 5th ed. Hoboken, NJ: John Wiley and Sons, Inc.

Franklin CA, Worgan JP, eds. [2005]. Occupational and residential exposure assessment for pesticides. Sussex, England: John Wiley and Sons, Ltd., pp. 2–3.

Geno PW, Camann DE, Harding HJ, Villalobos K, Lewis RG [1996]. Handwipe sampling and analysis procedure for the measurement of dermal contact with pesticides. Arch Environ Contam Toxicol 30(1):132–138.

NIOSH [1997a]. Hazard evaluation and technical assistance report: United States Department of Agriculture, Plant Inspection and Quarantine Station, Miami, FL. By Kiefer M. Cincinnati, OH: U.S. Department of Health and Human Services, Centers for Disease Control and Prevention, National Institute for Occupational Safety and Health. NIOSH HETA Report No. 94-0353-2629.

NIOSH [1997b]. Hazard evaluation and technical assistance report: United States Department of Agriculture, Animal and Plant Health Inspection Service, Miami, FL. By Kiefer M. Cincinnati, OH: U.S. Department of Health and Human Services, Centers for Disease Control and Prevention, National Institute for Occupational Safety and Health. NIOSH HETA Report No. 96-0083-2628.

Petch PA (peter.a.petch@aphis.usda.gov) [2008]. APHIS Safety and Health Manual. Private e-mail message Srinivas Durgam (sdurgam@cdc.gov), February 1.

Rosen J [1998]. Inspection services. In: Stellman JM, ed. Encyclopedia of occupational health and safety. 4th ed. Vol. III, Geneva: International Labor Office, pp.101.3–101.5.

Sullivan JJ [1990]. Memorandum of May 9, 1990, from J.J. Sullivan, Division of Parasitic Diseases, National Center for Infectious Diseases, to M. Kiley, Office of Health and Safety, Centers for Disease Control, U.S. Department of Health and Human Services.

Sullivan JJ [2008]. Telephone conversation on March 7, 2008, between J.J. Sullivan, National Center for Zoonotic, Vector-Borne, and Enteric Diseases, and S. Durgam, Division of Surveillance, Hazard Evaluations and Field Studies, National Institute for Occupational Safety and Health, Centers for Disease Control and Prevention, U.S. Department of Health and Human Services.

APPENDIX A: METHODS

Pesticide Air Sampling

Air samples were collected on sorbent tubes containing Tenax® (750 milligram) placed between two polyurethane foam plugs using SKC PCXR4 air sampling pumps (SKC Incorporated, Eighty Four, Pennsylvania) calibrated at a flow rate of 4 liters per minute. The inlet port of the sampling pump was connected to the sampling media with Tygon® tubing. All air sampling pumps were calibrated before and after use. For PBZ samples, the sampling media was attached to the employees' lapels within their breathing zone, roughly defined as an area in front of the shoulders with a radius of 6 to 9 inches. All samples were extracted according to procedures described in EPA Method 3545 and analyzed by gas chromatography-mass spectroscopy according to EPA Method TO-10A [EPA 2009]. Chromatogram peaks for all the eluted chemicals were identified and their identities confirmed from the spectral library.

The LOD for Endosulfan sulfate was 3 µg/sample. The MDC was obtained by dividing the analytical LOD by the sample volume. Therefore, for a sample volume of 1.6 m^3, the MDC was 1.88 µg/m^3. The LOD for the remainder of the pesticides listed in Table B1 was 2 µg/sample. Therefore, the MDC for a sampling volume of 1.6 m^3 would be 1.25 µg/m^3.

Pesticide Surface Sampling

Surface wipe samples were collected using a commercially available 10 x 10-cm Sof-Wick® dressing sponge (Johnson and Johnson, Arlington, Texas) moistened with 10 milliliters of 100% isopropyl alcohol [Curwin et al. 2005]. The collection procedure was as follows: (1) identify the surface to be sampled and mark a 2 x 1-ft area; (2) don a pair of disposable nitrile gloves; (3) place wipe flat on surface and wipe using horizontal S-strokes, side-to-side so the entire surface is covered; (4) fold the exposed side of the wipe in and wipe the area with vertical S-strokes; (5) fold the wipe once more and wipe the area with horizontal S-strokes; and (6) fold the pad, exposed side in, and place in a sterile container. A new pair of disposable gloves was used for each surface wipe sample. All samples were analyzed by gas chromatography-mass spectroscopy according to EPA Method TO-10A, modified for the wipe media [EPA 2009]. Chromatogram peaks for all the eluted chemicals were identified and their identities confirmed from the spectral library. The analytical LOD for pesticides analyzed in surface wipe samples ranged from 0.4–0.7 µg/sample.

References

Curwin BD, Hein MJ, Sanderson WT, Barr DB, Heederik D, Reynolds SJ, Ward EM, Alavanaja MC [2005]. Urinary and hand wipe pesticide levels among farmers and nonfarmers in Iowa. J Expo Anal Environ Epidemiol 15(6):500–508.

EPA [2009]. EPA standardized analytical methods. Chemical methods query. [http://www.epa.gov/sam/searchchem.htm]. Date accessed: March 2010.

APPENDIX B: OCCUPATIONAL EXPOSURE LIMITS AND HEALTH EFFECTS

In evaluating the hazards posed by workplace exposures, NIOSH investigators use both mandatory (legally enforceable) and recommended OELs for chemical, physical, and biological agents as a guide for making recommendations. OELs have been developed by Federal agencies and safety and health organizations to prevent the occurrence of adverse health effects from workplace exposures. Generally, OELs suggest levels of exposure that most employees may be exposed up to 10 hours per day, 40 hours per week for a working lifetime without experiencing adverse health effects. However, not all employees will be protected from adverse health effects even if their exposures are maintained below these levels. A small percentage may experience adverse health effects because of individual susceptibility, a preexisting medical condition, and/or a hypersensitivity (allergy). In addition, some hazardous substances may act in combination with other workplace exposures, the general environment, or with medications or personal habits of the employee to produce health effects even if the occupational exposures are controlled at the level set by the exposure limit. Also, some substances can be absorbed by direct contact with the skin and mucous membranes in addition to being inhaled, which contributes to the individual's overall exposure.

Most OELs are expressed as a TWA exposure. A TWA refers to the average exposure during a normal 8- to 10-hour workday. Some chemical substances and physical agents have recommended STEL or ceiling values where health effects are caused by exposures over a short period. Unless otherwise noted, the STEL is a 15-minute TWA exposure that should not be exceeded at any time during a workday, and the ceiling limit is an exposure that should not be exceeded at any time.

In the United States, OELs have been established by Federal agencies, professional organizations, state and local governments, and other entities. Some OELs are legally enforceable limits, while others are recommendations. The U.S. Department of Labor OSHA PELs (29 CFR 1910 [general industry]; 29 CFR 1926 [construction industry]; and 29 CFR 1917 [maritime industry]) are legal limits enforceable in workplaces covered under the Occupational Safety and Health Act. NIOSH RELs are recommendations based on a critical review of the scientific and technical information available on a given hazard and the adequacy of methods to identify and control the hazard. NIOSH RELs can be found in the *NIOSH Pocket Guide to Chemical Hazards* [NIOSH 2005]. NIOSH also recommends different types of risk management practices (e.g., engineering controls, safe work practices, employee education/training, personal protective equipment, and exposure and medical monitoring) to minimize the risk of exposure and adverse health effects from these hazards. Other OELs that are commonly used and cited in the United States include the TLVs recommended by ACGIH, a professional organization, and the WEELs recommended by the American Industrial Hygiene Association, another professional organization. The TLVs and WEELs are developed by committee members of these associations from a review of the published, peer-reviewed literature. They are not consensus standards. ACGIH TLVs are considered voluntary exposure guidelines for use by industrial hygienists and others trained in this discipline "to assist in the control of health hazards" [ACGIH 2009]. WEELs have been established for some chemicals "when no other legal or authoritative limits exist" [AIHA 2009].

Outside the United States, OELs have been established by various agencies and organizations and include both legal and recommended limits. Since 2006, the Berufsgenossenschaftliches Institut für Arbeitsschutz (German Institute for Occupational Safety and Health) has maintained a database of international

OELs from European Union member states, Canada (Québec), Japan, Switzerland, and the United States available at http://www.dguv.de/bgia/en/gestis/limit_values/index.jsp. The database contains international limits for over 1250 hazardous substances and is updated annually.

Employers should understand that not all hazardous chemicals have specific OSHA PELs, and for some agents the legally enforceable and recommended limits may not reflect current health-based information. However, an employer is still required by OSHA to protect its employees from hazards even in the absence of a specific OSHA PEL. OSHA requires an employer to furnish employees a place of employment free from recognized hazards that cause or are likely to cause death or serious physical harm [Occupational Safety and Health Act of 1970 (Public Law 91–596, sec. 5(a)(1))]. Thus, NIOSH investigators encourage employers to make use of other OELs when making risk assessment and risk management decisions to best protect the health of their employees. NIOSH investigators also encourage the use of the traditional hierarchy of controls approach to eliminate or minimize identified workplace hazards. This includes, in order of preference, the use of: (1) substitution or elimination of the hazardous agent, (2) engineering controls (e.g , local exhaust ventilation, process enclosure, dilution ventilation), (3) administrative controls (e.g., limiting time of exposure, employee training, work practice changes, medical surveillance), and (4) personal protective equipment (e.g., respiratory protection, gloves, eye protection, hearing protection). Control banding, a qualitative risk assessment and risk management tool, is a complementary approach to protecting employee health that focuses resources on exposure controls by describing how a risk needs to be managed. Information on control banding is available at http://www.cdc.gov/niosh/topics/ctrlbanding/. This approach can be applied in situations where OELs have not been established or can be used to supplement the OELs, when available.

Pesticides

A pesticide is any substance or mixture intended to prevent, destroy, repel, or mitigate insects (insecticide, miticide, acaricide); rodents (rodenticide); nematodes (nematocide); fungi (fungicide); or weeds (herbicide) designated as a "pest." Each type of pesticide has numerous modes of action, chemical classes, target organs, formulations, and physicochemical properties. Pesticide toxicity is equally diverse, and even within a similar chemical class, individual compounds ranging from extremely toxic to practically nontoxic can be found. As such, generalizations about the toxicity of pesticides cannot be made without considerable qualification and explanation. In the United States, regulatory responsibility to protect public health and the environment from the risks posed by pesticides lies with the EPA Office of Pesticide Programs. In the United States alone, approximately five billion pounds of pesticide products are used each year [EPA 2001]. Table B1 contains the list of 20 pesticides we analyzed for in air and on surfaces and their relevant OELs.

Table B1. Pesticides and associated OELs

Pesticide	NIOSH REL	OSHA PEL	ACGIH TLV	NIOSH Carcinogenicity
		µg/m³		
4,4'-DDD*	500	1000	1000	
4,4'-DDE*	500	1000	1000	
4,4'-DDT	500	1000	1000	Ca†
Aldrin	250	250	250	Ca
BHC-alpha	500	500	500	
BHC-beta	500	500	500	
BHC-delta	500	500	500	
BHC-gamma	500	500	500	
Chlordane-alpha	500	500	500	Ca
Chlordane-gamma	500	500	500	Ca
Dieldrin	250	250	250	Ca
Endosulfan I	100	None	100	
Endosulfan II	100	None	100	
Endosulfan sulfate	None	None	None	
Endrin	100	100	100	
Endrin aldehyde	None	None	None	
Endrin ketone	None	None	None	
Heptachlor	500	500	50	Ca
Heptachlor epoxide	None	None	50	
Methoxychlor	LFC‡	15000	10000	Ca

* Isomers of 4,4'-DDT

† Considered a potential occupational carcinogen by NIOSH

‡ Lowest feasible concentration

References

ACGIH [2009]. 2009 TLVs® and BEIs®: threshold limit values for chemical substances and physical agents and biological exposure indices. Cincinnati, OH: American Conference of Governmental Industrial Hygienists.

AIHA [2009]. AIHA 2009 Emergency response planning guidelines (ERPG) & workplace environmental exposure levels (WEEL) handbook. Fairfax, VA: American Industrial Hygiene Association.

CFR. Code of Federal Regulations. Washington, DC: U.S. Government Printing Office, Office of the Federal Register.

EPA [2001]. Pesticides industry sales and usage. 2000 and 2001 market estimates. [http://www.epa.gov/oppbead1/pestsales/01pestsales/market_estimates2001.pdf]. Date accessed: March 2010.

NIOSH [2005]. NIOSH pocket guide to chemical hazards. Cincinnati, OH: U.S. Department of Health and Human Services, Centers for Disease Control and Prevention, National Institute for Occupational Safety and Health, DHHS (NIOSH) Publication No. 2005-149. [http://www.cdc.gov/niosh/npg/]. Date accessed: March 2010.

ACKNOWLEDGMENTS AND AVAILABILITY OF REPORT

The Hazard Evaluations and Technical Assistance Branch (HETAB) of the National Institute for Occupational Safety and Health (NIOSH) conducts field investigations of possible health hazards in the workplace. These investigations are conducted under the authority of Section 20(a)(6) of the Occupational Safety and Health Act of 1970, 29 U.S.C. 669(a)(6) which authorizes the Secretary of Health and Human Services, following a written request from any employer or authorized representative of employees, to determine whether any substance normally found in the place of employment has potentially toxic effects in such concentrations as used or found. HETAB also provides, upon request, technical and consultative assistance to federal, state, and local agencies; labor; industry; and other groups or individuals to control occupational health hazards and to prevent related trauma and disease.

The findings and conclusions in this report are those of the authors and do not necessarily represent the views of NIOSH. Mention of any company or product does not constitute endorsement by NIOSH. In addition, citations to websites external to NIOSH do not constitute NIOSH endorsement of the sponsoring organizations or their programs or products. Furthermore, NIOSH is not responsible for the content of these websites. All Web addresses referenced in this document were accessible as of the publication date.

This report was prepared by Srinivas Durgam and Carlos Aristeguieta of HETAB, Division of Surveillance, Hazard Evaluations and Field Studies. Analytical support was provided by Bureau Veritas North America. Health communication assistance was provided by Stefanie Evans. Editorial assistance was provided by Ellen Galloway. Desktop publishing was performed by Robin Smith.

Copies of this report have been sent to employee and management representatives at USDA APHIS, the state health department, and the Occupational Safety and Health Administration Regional Office. This report is not copyrighted and may be freely reproduced. The report may be viewed and printed at http://www.cdc.gov/niosh/hhe/. Copies may be purchased from the National Technical Information Service at 5825 Port Royal Road, Springfield, Virginia 22161.

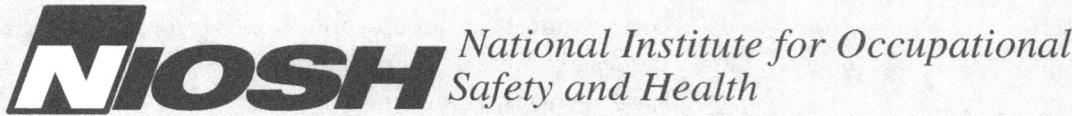

National Institute for Occupational Safety and Health

Delivering on the Nation's promise: Safety and health at work for all people through research and prevention.

To receive NIOSH documents or information about occupational safety and health topics, contact NIOSH at:

1-800-CDC-INFO (1-800-232-4636)

TTY: 1-888-232-6348

E-mail: cdcinfo@cdc.gov

or visit the NIOSH web site at: **www.cdc.gov/niosh.**

For a monthly update on news at NIOSH, subscribe to NIOSH eNews by visiting **www.cdc.gov/niosh/eNews.**

SAFER • HEALTHIER • PEOPLE™